WHY SLEEP IS ESSENTIAL

How Does The Peaceful Sleep Affect All Of Us?

20 Practical Ways To Improve Your Sleep

Andrew Simmones

TABLE OF CONTENTS

INTRODUCTION

'Sleep is the best meditation.'- Dalai Lama

Just as you need oxygen to breathe and food to stay nourished, you require sleep to stay fit, healthy and happy and function well. While many people think the body shuts down when we sleep, in reality, sleep is one of the most important processes occurring in our body throughout the day. This is not just your body and mind's way of getting rest and rejuvenating for another round of activity and work the next day, but sleep is actually the time when several important processes take place inside your system.

Irrespective of the fact that sleep is essential for your healthy functioning and wellbeing, many people disregard its importance and don't give their body enough rest on a regular basis. Many of us have the bad habit of sleeping anywhere from 3 to 5 hours at night on average and then waking up feeling groggy and leave straight for work.

This has been our routine for a long time and then we complain about low productivity, grumpy mood, anger management problems, lack of strength, inability to fulfill targets and goals and relationship problems.

While you may not realize this right now, a lack of sufficient sleep is one of the root causes behind all these problems, and if you wish to live a good quality life, you need to work on improving your sleeping habits.

If you agree on this and wish to sleep better, you have landed at the right spot. This book provides insight into the many reasons why getting a good night's sleep and ample rest is substantial for your wellbeing and survival, and provides 20 practical ways to improve your sleep routine and habits.

CHAPTER 1: UNDERSTANDING SLEEP AND ITS STAGES

Sleep is that one beautiful phase wherein you bid adieu to the world and drift off in your own world of dreams and sometimes not even that, and just relax. However, there is a lot more to sleep than just this and if you wish to sleep better, it is important you understand the different stages of sleep so you know exactly how you have been sleeping all this while.

Stages of Sleep

Before the invention of the electroencephalograph (EEG), scientists could not study sleep in detail. It was after this invention that they dug deeper into sleep and its different stages. There are two main kinds of sleep: NREM (non-rapid eye movement) which is also referred to as 'quiet sleep' and REM (rapid eye movement) which is referred to as 'paradoxical' or 'active' sleep.

When you sleep, you are quite alert and awake for some time. At that time, your brain functions in the beta waves that are rapid, fast and have short wavelengths. These brainwaves produces alertness, which is why you can still hear things around you actively and feel somewhat awake when you just drift off to sleep. It takes your brain 10 to 20 minutes and sometimes even longer to slow down and unwind.

As your brain relaxes, it produces alpha waves that are slower and have longer wavelength. These brainwaves also create calmness in the body, which is why you feel relaxed after a few hours of sleeping. However, even during this phase, you aren't in deep sleep. This is time when you can experience vivid and even strange sensations referred to as 'hypnagogic hallucinations' such as feeling like someone is calling out to you, or falling down in a deep pit etc. Another commonly occurring experience during this phase is the 'myoclonic jerk', which is feeling, startled for no apparent reason.

Let us take a deeper look into the different stages of sleep.

- NREM Phase 1: This is the phase when you have just fallen asleep and are relatively in light sleep. This is mostly considered as the transitioning period between deep sleep and wakefulness. In this stage, high amplitude waves 'theta waves' are produced that are slow brain waves. This phase lasts for 5 to 10 minutes mostly and if you are woken up during this phase, you may not recall drifting off to sleep.

- NREM Phase 2: During this phase, you become less aware of the happenings in your surrounding environment, your body temperature drops a little and your heartbeat and breathing becomes regular. This stage lasts for around 20 to sometimes 30 minutes and this is when your brain creates bursts of rhythmic brain wave activity, which is referred to as 'sleep spindles.' As per the American Sleep Foundation, we spend around half of our total sleep time in this phase.

- NREM Phase 3: In this stage, your brain produces delta waves which are slow, deep brainwaves which is why this phase is also at times known as 'delta sleep.' Your body relaxes in this stage and you become relatively less responsive to your surroundings and the noises as well as activities in it as compared to the first two stages. This is the transitional stage between light and extremely deep sleep. Your muscles relax and breathing rate and blood pressure drop in this stage. Sleep walking mostly occurs during this stage.

- REM Stage: This is the stage wherein your brain becomes quite active as compared to the other 3 stages. Your body becomes immobilized as it is extremely relaxed and your eyes move rapidly, which is a sign of you having dreams. Mostly, dreams occur during this very stage along with an increased brain activity and respiration rate. As per the American Sleep Foundation, on average we spend about 20% of our total sleep time in this stage. This stage is also known as 'paradoxical sleep' because your muscles become extremely relaxed in this stage as the voluntary muscles are immobilized whereas your brain and the rest of the systems become quite active.

An important thing to understand is that your sleep does not progress smoothly from phase 1 to 4 in a sequential manner. Sleep starts at stage 1 and then shifts into stage 2 followed by stage 3. Once again, you move back to stage 2 and then you enter REM sleep. Once this stage ends, you return to stage 2 and then wake up. Your sleep cycles through all these stages in this sequence about 4 to 5 times throughout the time you are asleep.

On average, it takes us 90 minutes to enter REM phase once we drift off to sleep. The first REM sleep cycle lasts for a short time, but it becomes longer with each cycle and tends to last for an hour. This brings us to an important question- how much sleep do we really need?

Our Sleep Requirements

Healthy and adequate sleep is important for everyone, but how much is adequate you may ask. Our sleep requirement decreases as we age. Infants and toddlers need anywhere from 12 to 16 hours of sleep but as they start going to school, their sleep requirement decreases to 11 to 14 hours. Children between 4 and 12 years of age need about 9 to 12 hours of sleep and teenagers require 8 to 10 hours of sleep on average. Adults too require the same amount of sleep, but mostly require 7 to 9 hours of well-rested sleep to function well daily.

You need to get enough sleep according to your age's requirement for your optimal alertness, development, growth and wellbeing. Sadly, you cannot accumulate sleep deprivation for some time and then stock up on hours of sleep to neutralize its effect. It doesn't work that way which is why you need to focus on getting at least 7 to 9 hours of sleep at night daily followed by 10 to 60 minutes of nap time during the day to function properly.

Now that you are clear on what stages constitute your sleep and how much hours of sleep you must get, let us move on to the next chapter to find out the importance of getting adequate sleep.

Chapter 2: The Importance Of Having Adequate Sleep

'Early to bed, early to rise makes a man healthy, wealthy and wise.'- Benjamin Franklin

What Benjamin Franklin said years ago is indeed true. Even science has proven that those who sleep and rise early and get a good night's rest tend to be happier and more successful in life as compared to those who miss out on a good night's sleep on a regular basis. Let us dig deeper into the importance of sleeping well by listing out the many reasons why you must build a healthy sleep routine:

Provides Your Body with Enough Rest and Improves Your Energy Levels

Sleep is the time when your body relaxes after a full day of toil and your worked out and torn muscles get to rejuvenate during that time. This is the time when different growth hormones are also released in your body to repair the worn out muscles and rehabilitate them. If you keep pushing your body to work throughout the night as well and that too on a regular basis, it explains why you feel so exhausted always.

Not only your body, but your mind also needs to rest after an entire day of thinking actively. The truth is, your mind is still working when you rest and sleep, but the activity does slow down and it works on areas other than analytical thinking, planning, brainstorming and active decision-making, which gives it a chance to unwind and relax.

This explains why you find it easier to comfortably leave your bed and feel fresh after a good night's rest. According to a survey by the 'Better Sleep Council', 32% Americans believe that one of the best benefits of getting a solid's night rest is their increased physical and mental energy. Sufficient sleep helps stabilize the hormones in your body, which also helps you make healthier eating choices. This consequently steadies the sugar levels in your body, which provides you with sustained energy throughout the day.

Improves Your Heart Health and Blood Pressure

If you are worried of having poor heart health since it runs in your family, start improving your sleep routine. A study shows that a solid night's sleep is a great way to safeguard your heart against cardiac arrest. The study examined the sleep habits of over 52,000 Norwegian people and observed that those who sleep less and experience insomnia have a 30 to 45% greater risk of experiencing a heart attack as compared to those who sleep well throughout the night. A lack of sleep often leads to high blood pressure as well as hormonal changes in your body, both of which pave way for a cardiac arrest. When you sleep well, these issues resolve and your heart health improves which then reduces your likelihood of experiencing heart related problems.

Also, studies show people who get less sleep have 80% more chances of experiencing hypertension (high blood pressure) than those who sleep properly through the night. Deep sleep helps stabilize your blood pressure as it lowers down during that time. This regulates your heartbeat and blood pressure, which helps you overcome hypertension.

Improved Emotional Wellbeing

It should not come as a surprise to you that sleeping well does cheer you up. Compare your mood and emotional wellbeing when you sleep well through the night to a time when you keep tossing and turning on your bed the entire night. The answer shows a marked improvement in your cheerfulness and your ability to think clearly.

Ample sleep improves the production of mood improving hormones such as serotonin and dopamine, which boost your confidence, energy, and happiness helping you stay energetic, happy, calm and enthusiastic throughout the day.

Also, when you feel happy, you stay positive, which improves your ability to think clearly and make rational decisions. A study by the National Sleep Foundation also shows that there exists a strong and complicated association between depression and insomnia. People suffering from insomnia have a 10 times more likelihood of suffering from depression as compared to the healthy sleepers. One reason behind this is that often when you don't sleep, you rehash the past memories or think about the future concerns which can often open old wounds or make you too concerned about the future, respectively. This increases your tensions and paves way for depression.

Fortunately, these issues can be combatted successfully especially by improving your sleep routine. When you rest properly through the night, you allow your body to stabilize the hormonal issues, which improves your mood and consequently the quality of your life.

Moreover, a survey by the National Sleep Foundation found out that over 85% participants of the study who received insufficient sleep throughout the night complained that this adversely affected their temper and mood; 72% reported that a lack of sleep impacts their household responsibilities and family life; and 68% stated that it negatively influenced their social lives. This happens because a lack of sleep also increases the levels of cortisol in your body, which is the notorious stress hormone. The more the cortisol in your body, the more you feel stressed out. That said, getting a good night's rest daily helps lower the cortisol levels and improves your mood.

Helps You Eat Healthy and Manage your Weight

If you are having a hard time managing your weight, pay attention to your sleep routine. It is likely you stay awake for the major part of the night and this is a major reason why you do not have healthy eating habits and cannot lose weight successfully.

Experts suggest that skipping sleep is often the culprit that keeps you from losing weight easily because it messes with your metabolism. People who do not sleep well mostly have low levels of 'leptin', which is the satiety hormone. Low levels of leptin means you feel satiated slowly and eat more to feel satisfied.

Also, a lack of sleep promotes the production of 'ghrelin' which is the hunger hormone so not sleeping enough means you feel hungrier throughout the day and eat more. This is why you are always feeling ravenous particularly for sugar-laden foods.

Studies show that healthy sleepers who get at least 6 to 8 hours of sleep on average are better able to follow their weight loss regimen primarily because their ghrelin and leptin levels are stabilized.

Also, since sleeping well increases your energy levels and ability to think rationally, you are able to feel fresher and make healthier food choices during the day and stay on the right track when it comes to losing weight.

Reduces Risk of Suffering from Diabetes

Inadequate sleep over a long period can make you develop high insulin resistance, which is a precursor to suffering from diabetes. Research has also discovered that the quality and duration of your sleep affect the levels of hormones involved in triggering diabetes; therefore, if you sleep less, you are likely to become more prone to acquiring diabetes or pre-diabetes. Improving your sleep routine is definitely a way to overcome these problems and stay fitter.

Reinforces Your Immune System

Research shows that healthy sleepers have a better immune system than the ones who complain of never sleeping enough. A study in Archives of Internal Medicine from 2009 shows that those who sleep fewer than 7 hours at night have 3 times more chances of suffering from common cold as compared to those who sleep longer than that. If you want a strong, healthy immune system that kicks off diseases efficiently from your system, have adequate sleep.

Improves Your Skin

Yes, 'beauty sleep' does exist and it is exactly what you need to have a healthy, supple and glowing skin. Restorative, deep sleep improves the production of your body cells, which reduces the breakdown of skin proteins and helps your skin repair the damage it goes through which improves its health and condition.

Improves Your Love Life and Relationships

Studies show that when you sleep less, you become more irritable towards your partner and even everyone else during the day, which only negatively affects your relationships.

In addition, a lack of sleep makes you grumpy, stressed out and annoyed which decreases your ability to stay calm with people and make better decisions. This does take a toll on your love life and other important relationships.

Fortunately, this can be reversed by improving your sleep routine. Healthy sleepers tend to have a better marriage and build healthy relationships in life as compared to insomniacs as the former are more composed, calmer, energetic and happier in life.

A study in 2011 shows that improved sleep also improves your sex drive and consequently your sex life. This can be because a good night's rest improves your energy levels and enthusiasm. Also, it boosts testosterone levels in men, which improves their libido. Therefore, when you sleep well daily, you are likely to enjoy better sex life with your partner, which also improves your love/ marital life.

Improved Brainpower

A healthy sleep routine does wonders to your brainpower. A deep REM sleep helps reinforce the important pieces of information you noticed during the day and crates long-term memories.

Further, during your sleep, your brain discards meaningless information from your mind to prevent information overload. Your brain also clears out toxins out of your system when you are asleep, which improves your brain health and overall cognition.

Additionally, a good night's rest improves your brain's plasticity and connectivity. Plasticity is required for improved learning and reinforcing your memory. There is plenty of evidence, which suggests how a lack of sleep can cause problems with your working memory and hampers your ability to process information. If you wish to have a sharper memory and improved cognition, just focus on getting enough sleep.

Reduces Likelihood of Acquiring Cancer

A study in the journal titled 'Cancer' discovered that those who sleep 6 or fewer hours at night have a staggering 50% risk of acquiring colorectal adenomas which is a precursor to having cancerous tumors as compared to all those who clock in at a minimum of 7 hours every night. Another study shows that a lack of sleep increases your chances of suffering from colon cancer.

Improves Your Focus and Productivity

Naturally, when you rest well, you focus better on your work, which improves your work performance and reduces slip-ups. This increases your productivity and opens up more opportunities of growth and advancement in your career so you can easily accomplish your professional goals.

All these positive changes in your life help you live better and feel good about yourself. Also, a study published in 2007 shows that adequate sleep helps you cope successfully with chronic pain as it relaxes your joints and muscles and improves your ability to manage pain.

Now that you are aware of all the reasons why you MUST SLEEP WELL, let us share with you the ways you can implement to improve your sleep routine.

Chapter 3: Improve Your Sleep Environment

Your environment plays a monumental role in affecting your different behaviors, decisions, moods and life in general. This holds truth for your sleep routine as well. If your sleep environment aka your bedroom is not conducive to a good night's rest, that maybe the reason why you do not sleep well at night. Here are a few practical changes you can bring to your sleep environment today to start sleeping better:

1. Dim the Lights in the Room before Going to Bed

Studies show that a dark environment actually helps trigger your sleep faster than one with glaring lights. If you sleep with all the lights switched on in your room, dim them a little now. Keep one low light on when you hit the bed to sleep as a dark environment relaxes your brain and activates the alpha waves. These slow, calm waves help you unwind and initiate sleep quickly.

Also, invest in blackout shades and heavy curtains to block out light coming in your room from the windows so you do not wake up before your rising time and sleep well throughout the night.

2. Check the Room Temperature

If your room is too hot or too cold, that maybe the reason why you keep tossing and turning on your bed the entire night. You cannot sleep when you feel hot or even when your toes are too cold. Experts suggest that temperatures between 60 and 75 degrees Fahrenheit during the summers are good enough to enable you to sleep well.

If you live in a hot country or during the summer season, make sure, your room is well ventilated so you don't feel too hot and wake up feeling exasperated. Also, invest in an efficient cooling and heating system that keeps the temperature of your house well regulated year around promoting a good night's sleep.

When it is hot, use a fan or air conditioner to keep the air nice and cool and if you can open a window, please do to allow fresh air into the room.

As for the chilly winters, keep your room warm enough so you stay cozy throughout your sleep. Use a central heating system to regulate the room's temperature, wear a couple of layers and use a comfy blanket to stay warm during your sleep.

3. Keep Your Room Calm and Quiet

If you sleep in a noisy, room or have loud noises coming in your room during the night; that explains why you fail to sleep well. Before going to bed, ensure you switch off all sorts of noisy appliances or anything that creates even a low but constant noise because that can really get to you while you sleep.

In addition, if you have noisy neighbors, request them to keep it down during the night. You can also invest in noise cancellation installations in your house walls to block noise coming off from the surroundings. Moreover, if you have a pet who has a habit of making loud noises throughout the night or at certain instances, keep him or her out of your room.

4. Invest in Comfy Bed, Mattress, Pillows and Bedspreads

Sometimes a hard bed or an uncomfortable mattress or pillows that are too high or a bedspread that feels itchy can keep you from drifting off to sleep easily at night. Pay close attention to your bed, mattress, pillows and bed sheets and if any of these feel uncomfortable to you, it is time to invest in some new, super comfortable ones.

Get a bed size according to your physique and sleep needs. If you like to move around on your bed and are plus size, and sleep alone, it is best to invest in at least a Queen size bed instead. However, if you and your partner sleep together, invest in a nice Queen or King size bed so both of you can sleep comfortably on it.

As for your mattress, it needs to properly support your spine and legs. If it feels too stiff against your bed or you completely fall inside it and it is too soft, you are likely to experience back problems in a while which will get in the way of your good night's rest. Replace the mattress with a nice, comfy one. If you want a mattress that offers pressure relief, body contouring and great spinal support, get a memory foam. However, if you want a nice bouncy mattress that is cool to sleep on and offers great comfort, a latex one may serve you well.

Similarly, coiled mattress offer great support and bounce too, so you can purchase this if it suits your body well. However, some people also complain of experiencing back problems because of coiled mattresses and prefer latex ones to them. If you wish to have a softer bed, invest in a pillow top mattress as it comes with extra cushioning.

Moreover, make sure to buy nice, soft bed linen for your bed. Choose a material according to the season because certain materials work well only in certain seasons and can feel too warm in summers. For instance, silk and wool covers are suitable for winters whereas cotton is more appropriate for summers, but works fine year around as well.

As for your pillow, it needs to be just 3 to 4 inches in height and must be soft enough for you to lie on. If it is too hard, it may be the culprit behind your stiff neck and constant headaches and obviously a lack of sleep. Bring these changes to your bed and you are likely to snooze easily.

5. Leverage the Power of Natural Light

Natural light is a great way to improve your sleep-wake cycle and keeps your internal clock ticking off healthily. If there is no adequate light in your room, that maybe another reason why you have an unhealthy sleep-wake cycle and sleep as well as wake up at odd hours.

While it is important to close the blinds when going to sleep, keep one slightly open so you allow natural light to flow in when the sun rises and leverage its power to help you wake up comfortably. With time, this will improve your sleep-wake cycle allowing you to sleep early and rise on time as well.

6. Change the Position of Your Bed

The position of your bed too plays quite a role in determining the quality of your sleep. If it is right next to the door and your partner keeps waking up throughout the night to move in and out of the room or has a sleep routine and work timings different from yours, it can be the reason why you have interrupted sleep daily.

Also, if your bed is close to the wall adjacent to the kitchen or a noisy room or right in front of a large window in your room, it can be another reason why you fail to sleep well at night. Naturally, when noise keeps disturbing you while you struggle to sleep or a huge gush of light falls on your face early in the morning, way before your rising time, you are unable to sleep.

In these cases, it is best to change the position of your bed and move it to a quieter nook in your room to sleep better. As you bring these changes to your sleep environment, make a few to your sleep routine and habits to promote better sleep at night.

CHAPTER 4: IMPROVE YOUR SLEEP ROUTINE AND HABITS

All of us have certain sleeping habits that we engage in before going to bed. Often, these habits affect the duration and quality of our sleep. Let us look at the healthy sleep routine and related habits you need to build to allow your body to get ample rest throughout the night:

7. Reduce Your Exposure to Blue Light in the Evening

While it is crucial to expose yourself to natural light during the day time to improve your internal clock, it is crucial to limit your exposure of blue light in the evening and nighttime. Blue light, mostly emitted by electronic devices such as computers, iPads and smartphones adversely affects your circadian rhythm which makes you brain feel that it is still day time.

When your brain gets this wrong signal, it signals your body to decrease the production of melatonin, which is an important hormone involved in your sleep. It helps you unwind and enjoy deep, restorative sleep.

Naturally, when there is less of melatonin in your body, you find it difficult to fall asleep and stay asleep throughout the night. To improve your sleep, make sure you reduce your exposure to blue light especially in the evening and night so your brain naturally feels the day has ended and you can doze off easily. Here are a few ways to do that:

- Stop using electronic devices especially your phone at least 2 hours before going to bed. This keeps blue light off your eyes and brain before your bedtime helping you unwind easily.

- Install apps on your phone and laptop that block the blue light such as f.lux.

- Try not to watch TV and dim bright lights 1 to 2 hours before going to sleep to promote a good night's rest.

8. Set Consistent Wake and Sleep Times

Your circadian rhythm functions on a consistent loop and aligns itself with the sunset and sunrise. This means that if you are consistent with your wake up and sleep times, you are able to sleep better.

A study even shows that people with irregular sleep routine reported having poor sleep. In addition, irregular sleep and wake up times negatively affect your melatonin levels in the body, which keeps you from sleeping well.

Set a specific sleep, wake up time, and make sure to hit the bed and wake up at those particular times strictly. First, observe how much sleep you need to feel fresh and active the next day. Try to keep your routine throughout the day the same for 3 to 5 days and sleep for 7, 8 and 9 hours over this time period. Observe your activity and performance levels on the days you slept for 7, 8 and 9 or even 10 hours and see what duration suits you most. Some people feel fresher sleeping for 9 hours whereas for some, sleeping for 7 hours is sufficient because sleeping for 9 hours makes them feel a little groggy.

Once you have figured out the duration of sleep you need to feel active and healthy, set a sleep and rising time accordingly. If you have to wake up at 6am so you can shower, change comfortably and have breakfast before leaving for work at 8:30am, make sure to hit the bed at around 10-11pm 10pm if you need 7 hours of sleep at night.

Once you settle on your sleep and wake up times, go to bed at that time daily even if you don't feel sleepy then or feel like going to bed an hour earlier that day. Don't mess with your circadian rhythm please. Also, set alarms to wake up exactly at 6 am even if you couldn't sleep well for a few days.

It takes your body a few days to adjust your circadian rhythm so be patient and give yourself enough time to settle in to the new routine. Soon, you will be sleeping like a baby throughout the night.

9. Reduce Longer and Irregular Naps in the Day

Napping in the day does help you function effectively and efficiently and improves your productivity. That said, if you nap for hours during the day or at irregular times, this again messes up your circadian rhythm keeping you from sleeping easily at night.

Depending on your sleep time, set a naptime at least 5 to 6 hours before it and do not nap for longer than an hour. This helps you drift off to sleep at your exact bedtime without feeling too active at night.

10. Create a Pre-sleep Routine

Mostly, people take a while to unwind and initiate sleep at night. An easier way to relax your stressed nerves is to create a nice pre-sleep routine that helps you unwind an hour or two before your bedtime so you sleep easily at the right time.

Do anything relaxing an hour or two before hitting the bed. According to studies, taking warm showers, reading a nice book, listening to soothing songs and massaging your body and head before sleeping relaxes your body and mind promoting a solid night's sleep. If there is anything else that calms you down, engage in that for a minimum of 60 minutes before sleeping. This also helps you create a nice ritual of spending some quality time with yourself, which improves your emotional wellbeing and when you feel calmer, you naturally sleep better.

In addition to incorporating these habits in your routine, also work on improving your lifestyle because a healthier lifestyle does promote a healthy sleep routine. The next chapter teaches you how to do that.

Chapter 5: A Healthier Lifestyle Leads To A Healthy Sleep Routine

If your lifestyle is not active and healthy, that is another reason why you do not get to enjoy enough sleep at night. Here are some improvements you can bring in your lifestyle to sleep better:

11. Say No to Caffeine in the Evening

While caffeine does benefit you, consuming it later in the day can stimulate your nervous system too much and make you active at night. A study shows that consuming caffeine even 6 hours before your bedtime worsens your sleep quality. Make sure only to have coffee in the morning and limit your intake of caffeinated beverages throughout the rest of the day so you sleep easily at night.

12. Reduce Fluid Intake Later in the Day

Drinking 8 to 10 glasses of water along with healthy fluids helps you stay hydrated and healthy, but increased fluid intake in the evening only fills up your bladder too quickly leading to frequent trips to the bathroom at night. The result: poor sleep quality! If you have a habit of drinking water or fluids throughout the day, make sure to limit their intake in the evening. Drink little to no water 1 to 3 hours before bedtime so your sleep isn't interrupted by the urge to empty your bladder.

13. Eat Lighter Meals in the Evening

Filling up your tummy with heavy meals tends to be satisfying, but doesn't do your digestive system and sleep cycle much good. It takes 3 to 4 hours for your digestive system to digest a meal and if it is actively working right before your sleep time, you can have trouble falling asleep. Try to keep your evening meals light so you can sleep easily.

14. Reduce Your Alcohol Consumption

Increased alcohol consumption messes up your circadian rhythm and the melatonin levels in your body, which obviously affects your sleep quality. If you consume too much alcohol regularly, slowly cut back on it to stay fit and sleep well.

15. Stay Active

A sedentary lifestyle is a huge reason why most people find it hard to sleep properly. If you do not exercise at all or engage in any physical activity and have a work routine that requires you to sit in front of the computer screen all day long, this is another reason why you have a hard time sleeping.

Whatever your work requirement is, ensure you stay active throughout the day. This improves your hormonal balance in your body making you drift off to bed easily.

16. Exercise Daily

In addition, ensure you exercise daily or at least 4 to 5 times a week for at least 15 to 60 minutes. This improves the production of serotonin, dopamine and melatonin, which improve your energy levels and sleep cycle helping you sleep well at night. Also, exercise makes your muscles work out and if you are active throughout the day and exercise, you feel exhausted by the time you hit the bed and sleep easily.

To exercise, choose any physical activity you enjoy such as swimming, jogging, Pilates or a sport etc. and engage in it alone or with a friend for 15 to 60 minutes daily. Start with 15 minutes and slowly increase the duration.

17. Exercise Early

While exercising helps you sleep well, make sure you don't exercise later in the day. Late evening or nighttime exercise makes you too enthusiastic and increases your energy levels, which can make it difficult for you to sleep at your bedtime. Ensure to exercise during the morning time, preferably 7 to 8 hours before your bedtime.

18. Eat Healthy

Several studies prove that a low fat or high carb diet is often the reason behind poor quality sleep. While a good amount of carbs is essential for your optimal growth and development, make sure to consume carbs earlier in the day. At night, eat meals low in carbs and high in fats as this too promotes better sleep.

19. Take Melatonin Supplements

Melatonin as you already know is essential for good quality sleep. In addition to working on the methods taught above to increase your melatonin levels, take a melatonin supplement for a few weeks to regulate its production in your body. Taking 1 to 5 mg of melatonin supplements 30 to 60 minutes before your bed time helps you sleep well and has no side-effects either. You can easily find them in good pharmacies. With time, as you start to sleep better, cut back and then eliminate your intake of these supplements.

20. Spend Time in Sunlight

Natural sunlight as you already know works well in stabilizing your circadian rhythm. To improve on that, spend some nice time in the sunlight, about 30 to 90 minutes daily, but make sure not to do so when the UV rays are at their peak, which is around 12 pm to 3 pm mostly.

Work consistently on these strategies and keep a record of what suits you well so you focus more on techniques that work out well in your favor.

CONCLUSION

As you have learned from this book, sleep is critical for healthy functioning of your body. If you have a difficult time falling and staying asleep, use the tips outlined in this book to sleep better and enjoy better rest, which will ensure that you function well when you are awake; thus, greatly increasing your productivity.

www.ingramcontent.com/pod-product-compliance
Lightning Source LLC
Chambersburg PA
CBHW072308170526
45158CB00003BA/1236